# Live Your Best Life as an Elder

## Finding the Senior Living Community for You

*By*
*Marian E. Karpisek*

# Table of Contents

# Dedication

In memory of my husband, Bob, and to my daughters, Kris Williams, and Jenny Storie; grandchildren: Aurora Storie, Brent Storie, Curt Storie, and Scott Sarka; my great-grandchildren: Jersey Young, Tanner Garnsey, Spencer Storie, Benson Storie, Everett Gryboski, Scarlet Storie, and Skyler Storie; my sister, Kathy Jones; and my sisters-in-law, Pat Weisberg and Shelly Edwards.

And, to my Pointe family. Thank you for your support and caring and for making my old age a very positive time in my life.

# Acknowledgments

This book would not have been possible without the support and help of many others. My husband, Bob, helped create the spreadsheet for assessing potential senior communities, and together, we visited sites and made our decision about where to live. Bob always encouraged me to pursue my goals and reach for what I wanted. He supported me fully in all my endeavors.

My sisters-in-law, Pat Weisberg and Shelly Edwards, provided tremendous hands-on support during the months Bob was in the hospital and care facilities. Without their help, I would not have survived as well as I have, and I certainly wouldn't have had the strength to write this book.

Kathy Jones, Jacque Turner and Beth Masterson read each chapter as I wrote it, critiqued it, and made very helpful suggestions. Their ideas were always right on and gave me direction and inspiration. The finished product would not have been as polished without their help.

Susan Rosenberg was invaluable as proofreader. Her eye for mistakes, wording, and meaning is impeccable.

My fellow residents provided much input through conversations and discussions about our lives in Independent Living. Their experiences provided a wider lens with which to view senior living in all its complexities.

# About the Author

Marian E. Karpisek is an active resident of a senior independent living community in Santee, California, where she has lived for almost four years. She has published four books and is currently the creator and editor of a newsletter, *Pointe of View,* published monthly for residents.

Born in Dover, Ohio, Marian graduated from Miami University with a B.S. in Ed. She earned her *M.S. in School Libraries* and an *Administrative Certificate* from the University of Utah. She retired as Library Supervisor for the Salt Lake City (UT) School District. She was also an Adjunct Professor of Library Science at Brigham Young University.

# How It All Began

## Introduction

My husband and I were 83 when we moved to an Independent Living community. Two years earlier, we had realized the time was not far off when we would no longer be able to live in our lovely townhouse. We had lived there for 20 years, and of all the houses we owned over our 61 years of marriage, it was our favorite.

The stairs were becoming more difficult for my husband. We only knew one of our neighbors well; we were two miles and a very steep hill from a shopping center, and public transportation didn't serve our small area. None of this boded well for our aging bodies.

At this point, we didn't know when we'd have to move, but knowing it was coming, we decided to explore senior communities to discover what was available for us. Except for visiting a few friends who had already made the move, we knew very little about what was involved or what would be important for us.

We had no real plan but began by making appointments and visiting a few of the senior communities close to our current home. The one thing we did, which proved to be exceptionally useful, was create a spreadsheet for comparing different sites. We had no idea what might be most important, just thoughts about what we might want.

This spreadsheet, much less complete than the one included in this book, proved to be extremely valuable as we spent two years looking at over 20 different communities. Some we dismissed immediately; others that we thought might work, we kept on file. When the time arrived and we knew it was time to move, we narrowed our search to four sites.

We went back to each and looked again, more closely. After this visit, we narrowed our field down to two and took our daughter with us for a third visit. Deciding on the one that seemed to best meet our needs, we made an appointment to sign a contract.

Despite being aware of the importance of contracts, we didn't think about getting a copy of the contract to study ahead of time, but our daughter did. We read it over carefully and marked a few areas where we had concerns. When the time came to sign, we were able to reach an agreement on our areas of concern.

We were pleased with our decision. We made new friends and became active in our community. I started a monthly newsletter, now in its fourth year, and we both participated in the many activities available.

Our new home wasn't perfect (no place will be), but we were happy and knew we had made the right choice. When my husband passed away, I realized, even more, how fortunate I am to live here. Not only do I have the support of my own family, but I also have the support of my senior living family.

While Bob was in the hospital and rehab for five months, I came home from visiting him to the warmth of my community. If I had been at my house, I would have gone home every night to an empty house and dinner on my own. Instead, I ate dinner with friends or, if I was tired, got take-out from the dining room and ate in my apartment. It was my choice, and no matter where I decided to eat, I didn't have to cook to have a good, nutritious dinner.

Friends and acquaintances in my building asked about Bob and how I was holding up. It was a good feeling to know so many others cared. The biweekly caregiver support group was a safe place where I could discuss how I was feeling with others who understood. And, after Bob passed, their support continued.

Since then, I have gotten to know several residents who initially moved to other communities and were disillusioned. They chose to move here and are much happier. Perhaps, if they had had a way to select a better fit, they would not have had to move.

Recently, I started thinking about how serendipitous our choice of a senior community was and how much easier our search would have been if we had known more. This book is intended to help you understand the options and parameters of searching for and finding a community that will be the best possible fit for you.

Marian Karpisek<br>
June, 2025<br>
Santee, California

# We're Getting Old! Is It Time To Move?

## Deciding Where to Spend Your Elder Years

As we reach our "elder years," many of us want to deny we're now officially "old," but it's time to look at reality! At some point, we must recognize the facts: we're not only seniors but elderly seniors!

"Traditionally, the 'elderly' are considered to be those persons age 65 and older. By that definition, in 1987, there were just over 30 million elderly people in the United States." [1] However, that definition doesn't reflect the new reality; many of us are still working, actively involved, and living full lives at 65. There is no exact age when we become "elderly." New research tentatively defines it as 78. [2]

Elders vary greatly in health, physical abilities, and mental acuity. Some of us, at age 78, are still traveling the world enthusiastically, others have become sedentary, while still others experience memory loss or serious medical issues. At some point, each of us knows deep inside, even if we don't admit it, that we're no longer the active go-getters we once were.

Even so, most of us would prefer to continue our "golden years" in our own homes for the rest of our days. In reality, that's often not the best place for us.

As our bodies slow down, we're not as agile as we once were. We're seeing more doctors, counting out pills, and feeling more aches and pains. We, and our friends, are getting knee and hip replacements, cataract surgery, hearing aids and dentures. Age creeps up on us, and we're finally forced to admit that our bodies are changing, and we need to consider some adjustments to where and how we live. This is one of the biggest issues as we age.

Most of us have lived in a residential neighborhood all our lives. We've never considered anything else and really don't want to change that scenario now. However, while we're still able, it's time to think seriously about our future.

If we wait too long to decide where we'll live and are mentally unable to make a decision for ourselves, our families may obtain legal guardianship, or a court-appointed conservator may have to make that decision for us.[3] It's much better to prepare before it's too late. By planning ahead, we have time to make our choices based on facts and priorities that will help us enjoy our lives as long as possible.

There are several options for where we may spend our remaining years. It's important to select the one that will give us the best quality of life, not only in the short term but also if we live to an advanced age. "The number of Americans ages 100 and older is projected to more than quadruple over the next three decades, from an estimated 101,000 in 2024 to about 422,000 in 2054, according to projections from the U.S. Census Bureau."[4]

We may decide we want to **stay in our current home** until we're carried out feet first. With enough help and adaptations to our home, this option is possible, but most often it's not the best long-term choice. We may decide to **live with a family member**. This may be a positive move if it's well thought out and planned, or it can be fraught with landmines that explode unexpectedly. We may consider a **55+ community designed for active seniors**. The fourth option is moving to a **senior living community**.

*When* is it time to start actively considering our options? Take the **Evaluation** survey to determine if you should consider a move as soon as possible or if you may have a year or more to research and find the best solution. Even if it looks like you can continue living in your home for the next few years, it's best to start planning and laying the groundwork now, so when the time comes for you to actually move, you'll be prepared.

## Interpreting Your Evaluation

After you've completed the **Evaluation**, look critically at your answers. Even if you're able to care for yourself and your home right now, the most important questions are those about your relationships.

*The National Institute of Health* reports that social isolation poses significant health risks. [5] If your answers indicate you don't have much interaction with others, it's time to seriously consider a move in the near future, regardless of your physical abilities.

## Options

### Continue to Live in Your Current Home for the Near Future

If your evaluation indicates you're doing well living alone, you're enjoying life, and have frequent social interactions with family and friends, continuing to live where you are at present is feasible. You're fortunate to have time to seriously plan for your future.

To stay comfortably in your current home, you may need to make some adaptations. Stairlifts, remodeled bathrooms, and ramps help accommodate your changing physical needs. Note that extensive renovations to your home may impact its future value, as buyers may not want these modifications.

You can hire assistance with personal needs as well. *Meals on Wheels* can bring two nutritious meals to you each day. Personal helpers can assist with dressing, bathing, and other daily tasks. A family member or someone with your Power of Attorney (*see Chapter 8*) may assist with financial issues and paying bills.

This help, however, may not be enough. Having helpers 24/7 is extremely expensive and takes time and energy to maintain. If you don't have the ability to handle this yourself, someone else will need to do it for you. And, although helpers provide companionship, it's not the same as family and friends.

If you don't have 24/7 helpers, you may spend large portions of your day alone, watching endless TV or being caught up in memories of the past. Being lonely, you become more vulnerable to scams. "Each year, millions of elderly Americans fall victim to some type of financial fraud or confidence scheme, including romance, lottery, and sweepstakes scams—just to name a few. Seniors are often targeted because they tend to be trusting and polite. They also usually have financial savings, own a home, and have good credit—all of which make them attractive to scammers." [6]

Life is getting more complex. As our minds slow down a bit, the world we're dealing with becomes more complicated. Also, keep in mind that the more help you hire and/or the more modifications you make to your home, the higher your cost of living will be. But, most important of all, remaining in your home does not take into account the increasing loneliness that can plague you as you continue to age.

## Living with Family

Another choice that may come to mind is moving in with family members. This may be a good idea financially, but it's also likely to create problems within your family. It's important to thoroughly scrutinize the ramifications not only for you and the family where you'll live but for all members of your extended family.

Location, finances, accessibility, and family support all must be considered. How much privacy will you have? How will your presence change the dynamics of the family? Will you be home alone all day while everyone else is off at work or school? How will this improve your situation?

Moving back and forth between family members is not recommended. You never feel completely at home anywhere, and you're essentially "living out of a suitcase." Your opportunity to make new friends is limited. Although this spreads the responsibility for your care among two or more of your children or other relatives, their lives are also in constant flux.

## Senior Apartments/Housing Developments (55 Plus Communities)

Senior housing developments are usually restricted to those 55 years and older. The homes may have adaptations such as no stairs and grab bars.[7] There may be a community center with an extensive menu of activities, or there may only be an occasional holiday potluck.

This type of housing may be ideal for younger seniors who are still in an active, healthy time of life. Neighbors are of a similar age, and most have moved to continue their active lives. However, usually, there are no support services such as transportation, meals, or on-site access to medical assistance.

## Senior Living Communities

Senior Living communities provide individual apartments and/or individual small cottages designed to meet the needs of residents. There are services and activities readily available to make your life easier and keep you actively involved with others. The remainder of this book will focus on senior Independent Living and Assisted Living communities, as these are the primary entry points for senior living.

## Summary

We can either go into our elder years fighting to retain life as it has been, or we can look at options for creating a new life responsive to our current and future needs. It takes courage to consider a major change in our lives when we would prefer our lives just continue on in the future as they have in the past. But, realistically, most of us don't have that option. If we don't make the decision of where we want to live and we become unable to do so, a guardian or conservator may have to make it for us, and their selection may not be the choice we would prefer.

# Evaluate Your Current Life
## Work Sheet

**Your Health:**

| | | | |
|---|---|---|---|
| How good is your overall health? | Excellent | Okay | Poor |
| Have you fallen in the last six months? | How Often? | _____ | |
| Do you have chronic health problems? | Yes | No | |
| Do you manage your own medications? | Yes | No | |
| Do you manage your own health appointments? | Yes | No | |
| How do you get to your medical appointments? | _____ | | |
| Do you use any assistive devices? | Cane | Walker | Wheelchair |

**General:**

| | | |
|---|---|---|
| Is there good public transit nearby? | Yes | No |
| Are stores and services close by? | Yes | No |
| Do you have helpful neighbors? | Yes | No |
| What outside personal help do you currently have or need? | List: | |

| | | |
|---|---|---|
| Do you have stairs? | Yes | No |
| If you have stairs, can you use them easily? | Yes | No |
| Do you have to pause for breath when | Yes | No |
| Can you bring groceries and other packages into your home easily? | Yes | No |
| Is your laundry room convenient? (Washer/dryer, folding clothes, hanging clothes, supply storage, etc.) | Yes | No |
| Is it easy to take laundry to and from the laundry room? | Yes | No |
| Is your kitchen convenient? | Yes | No |
| Is it easy to cook meals? | Yes | No |
| Who keeps your home clean? | I/we do | Someone else |

| | All | Some rooms | Part |
|---|---|---|---|
| How much of your home are you using? | All | Some rooms | Part |

| | | |
|---|---|---|
| Is your mail delivered to your door? | Yes | No |
| Do you have central heat and A/C? | Yes | No |
| Does your home need minor repairs? | Yes | No |
| Does your home need major repairs? | Yes | No |

**Your Outdoor Areas**

| | | |
|---|---|---|
| Who does your yard work? | I/we do | Someone else |
| Who takes care of trees, shrub cutting, weeding, mulching, etc.? | I/we do | Someone else |

| Who removes snow? | I/we do | Someone else | No snow |
|---|---|---|---|

## Your Car

| | | |
|---|---|---|
| Do you have a car? | Yes | No |
| Do you drive? | Yes | No |
| Are you comfortable driving? | Yes | No |
| Who arranges maintenance and insurance? | I/we do | Someone else |
| How old is your car? | Year: _____ | |
| Where do you park your car? | Garage/carport | Driveway | Street |

## Weather

| | | |
|---|---|---|
| Do you live in an area subject to extreme weather, hurricanes, wildfires, or tornadoes? | Yes | No |
| Do you have family close by who help? | Yes | No |

## Relationships

| | | |
|---|---|---|
| Do you have a family member living with you in your home? | Yes | No |
| Do you have family close by who help? | Yes | No |
| How often do you interact with family members? | Daily | Weekly | Occasionally |

| | | | |
|---|---|---|---|
| Do you count on family members to help you? | | Yes | No |
| How often do you interact with friends? | Daily | Weekly | Occasionally |
| Do your friends help you? | | Yes | No |
| If yes, are they older or younger than you? | | Older | Younger |
| Are you active in a religious community? | | Yes | No |
| Do you socialize with your neighbors? | | Yes | No |
| Do your neighbors help you out? | | Yes | No |
| Have you ever used paid caregivers? | | Yes | No |
| Do you belong to any clubs? | | Yes | No |
| Are you still working? | Full time | Part-time | Retired |

**Activities and hobbies** (Circle all that apply):

| | | | | |
|---|---|---|---|---|
| Movies | Concerts | Theater | Eating Out | Hiking |
| Walking | Swimming | Games | Music | Sports |
| Reading | Exercising | Fishing | Arts and Crafts | |
| Sewing | Collecting | List Others: | | |

# Finding the Best Fit for You

## All Senior Living Communities Are Not Alike!

Senior Living Complexes, no matter where they are located or what they look like, have similarities but very important differences. The fee structure, ownership of the community, levels of care, and federal and state laws are all important considerations when you're choosing a community. We'll look at each of these areas in more detail to help you choose the type of community that makes the most sense for you.

# Fee Structures

There are two basic fee structures, Continuing Care Retirement Communities (CCRCs) and Month-to-Month Lease Communities. Although the day-to-day amenities provided are similar, the financial structures are very different. Before choosing a community, it's important to know not just what the immediate costs will be but also what you can project to spend over the remainder of your life.

## Continuing Care Retirement Communities (CCRCs)

CCRCs (also known as "Life Plan Communities") require an initial lump sum payment upon contracting with the community. The amount of this payment varies greatly depending on the ownership of the community and where it's located. Nonprofit CCRCs, such as those owned by religious or fraternal organizations, usually have lower buy-in fees.

These entry fees vary greatly, ranging from $40,000 to more than $2,000,000.[8] The biggest benefit of selecting a CCRC is that you can't outlive your money. You will be taken care of as long as you live, even if your bank account runs dry. A CCRC also permits residents to remain within their community regardless of any, and all, declines in health.

In addition to the initial payment, there is a monthly fee to cover ongoing expenses such as utilities, meals, transportation, and activities. This fee may not increase at all over the remainder of your life or increase minimally when higher levels of care are required. This is important information to know before signing a contract.[9]

Most CCRCs have at least four levels of care: Independent Living, Assisted Living, Memory Care and Continuing Care, all usually found on the same campus. None of us wants to move to the higher levels of care, even when our physical condition makes it essential, but moving is a little easier when friends and acquaintances are found at the new residence.

CCRCs may specify a part of the down payment that will be refunded to heirs after the death(s) of the person or persons with the contract. This is appealing to those who want to ensure their heirs will inherit some portion of their life savings.

Unfortunately, some CCRCs have declared bankruptcy[10], leaving residents nowhere to live and no access to the part of their down payment that was supposed to revert to their heirs. This is not a common occurrence. It is important to check with your financial advisor about the viability of the community owner, their financial history, and how a loss would impact your long-range financial plan.

## Month-to-Month Leases

Senior Living Complexes with month-to-month leases usually have at least two levels of care, Independent Living and Assisted Living, although many also have Memory Care and some have Continuing Care. Unlike a CCRC, as care needs increase, the monthly rent increases substantially to cover the additional staff and services required.

A month-to-month contract gives the resident the flexibility to leave at any time by giving a one-month notice. Conversely, the owner of the facility may also ask residents to leave, for cause, with a month's notice. The specifics should be spelled out in the signed contract.

Increases in rent can be expected as the cost of living rises. Knowing the percentage of increases over the last five years and the percent of increases your state permits is important. Although the current rent may fit well within your budget, you need to know if your retirement income and investments will continue to support future rent increases and the possible need for more intensive care as you continue to age. As people living in a retirement community tend to live longer[11], it is better to plan for a long life. (One of the advantages of being our age is we're no longer afraid of dying young!)

## Additional Fees

In addition to the above-discussed costs, there often is an additional one-time fee, designated as a "Community Fee" or "Entry Fee." These one-time charges are for updating the apartment so it looks new and covering administration costs of the move-in. If, at any time, a resident moves to a different apartment in the same building, this fee, or a part of it, maybe charged again.

# Ownership

## Corporations

Many senior communities are owned by corporations. A corporation may own a single complex or have multiple sites in multiple states. Corporations may advertise lofty ideals, and they may fulfill them, but their primary purpose is making a profit.

There are advantages to living in a community owned by a corporation. Identical or similar floor plans, modified to meet climate and terrain issues, have been refined to reflect the design most useful for residents and staff. Corporations may purchase equipment, furnishings, and food in bulk through system-wide contracts, keeping costs down.

Staff positions, job descriptions, and training are systemized for maximum efficiency. Activities may vary from location to location based on community interests, but budgets for these will be set by the corporation.

However, it is more difficult to address and negotiate issues or problems that arise in an individual location when dealing with the corporate structure. The ability to address concerns at the local level may be more difficult as decisions may need to be made at a higher level.

## Single Owner

A senior complex may have a single owner or a local group dedicated to providing a service for an area with a need for senior housing. The advantage here is that the owners may be more closely connected to the community and, as a result, be more responsive to the needs of residents. They may have more of a hands-on approach to operating the facility and may be more open to suggestions from residents.

As long as the original concept remains in place, all can go well for residents. Problems may arise if the original owners decide to sell their facility to a corporation or turn it over to a management company. Significant changes can result that may or may not please the residents.

A single owner, having success with a single entity, may decide to build more facilities, and what was once a small independent operation can become part of something bigger with less of a personal connection. As the number of units increase, the layers of communication may make getting a timely response more difficult.

## Non-Profit Entities

Non-profit senior living communities are run by 501(c)(3)[12] non-profit organizations. Federal guidelines detail rules under which they must function and how any earnings must be spent. None of the organization's earnings can benefit any private shareholder or individual.[13]

These Senior living complexes may be owned by religious, professional, or ethnic groups whose mission is their focus rather than profit. Residency may be limited to those who qualify as part of the group or be open to anyone.

## U.S. Government

Section 202 Supportive Housing for the Elderly provides affordable housing options for "very low-income seniors" who are at least 62 years old and qualify. Although designed for independent living, the facility may offer support services such as cleaning, transportation, and cooking.[14]

The rent in a Supportive Housing community is 30% of adjusted income. Making less than 50% of the Area Median Income is required for acceptance.[15]

Section 202 housing for the elderly is secure and accessible for those with a variety of abilities and will have ramps, grab bars, wide doorways for wheelchairs, and non-slip surfaces. Reducing social isolation is a goal and there are common areas and recreational activities to bring residents together. Most of these communities are centrally located with nearby health services, shopping, and public transportation available.[16]

Apartments tend to be on the smaller side but include essentials for living, including a kitchen with all basic appliances, heating and A/C, storage space, and handicapped bathroom accessibility. There will be community areas, an on-site manager and recreational space.

In many areas of the country, this housing is in great demand, and there are years' long waiting lists. If you believe you may qualify for this type of housing, start doing your homework and get on the waiting list.

## Military

Military Veterans may find Assisted Living and Nursing Home facilities through the Veterans' Association (VA). This option is not open to the general public but may be a lifeline for those who meet the criteria.

To qualify, you must be enrolled in the VA health care system. They will evaluate your needs and decide if the service is necessary. There must be available space in a facility near where you live. Other factors may include service-connected disability status and insurance coverage. If you believe you may qualify, you can get more information by calling 877-222-8387, Monday through Friday, 8:00 a.m. to 8:00 p.m. E.T.[17]

# Levels of Care

There are six levels of care identified by *US News Health*.[18] They are:

- Independent Living

- Assisted Living

- Memory Care

- Custodial Care

- Skilled Nursing Care

- Short-term Care/Rehabilitation

Most month-to-month senior living complexes offer Independent Living and Assisted Living. Many additionally have Memory Care, and a smaller number also have Continuing Care. CCRC communities will normally have four levels of care; Independent Living, Assisted Living, Memory Care, and Continuing Care. Skilled nursing may be available in some communities.

In this book, we'll focus on the first two options: Independent Living and Assisted Living. This is where we opt to enter a senior living complex, and many of us will never use the higher levels of care, or if we do, it will be for short periods of time following a hospitalization. However, it's important to know what the higher levels of service provide even though we don't currently need them and hope to never need them.

Residents can enter senior living at the level of care needed at any time. Management may determine the level of care through an in-house assessment or a doctor's evaluation (usually required for Memory Care).

As availability at any level is often an issue, it is best to start searching available communities before the need is critical. Advanced planning and getting on a waiting list make it easier to proceed when the time arrives.

## Independent Living

Independent living is intended for seniors who can take complete care of themselves. They do not need assistance with the basic necessities of life but want to enjoy life without the responsibilities of a traditional home. Those using a walker or wheelchair may live in independent living if they do not require the facility to provide assistance.

Senior living housing may take the form of an apartment in a large building or individual cottages with access to the services of the greater community. Units usually have a living room, kitchen, one or two bedrooms, one or two bathrooms and house one or two residents. These complexes provide freedom from many responsibilities that come with living in a house or apartment. Additional services provided are meals, transportation, social and educational activities, and access to higher levels of care as needed.[19]

Residents of Independent Living come and go at will. If they still drive, they may continue many of their previous activities in the community at large. For those who no longer drive, transportation provided by the facility is available, and there is always *Uber, Lyft* or one of the many transportation services available for seniors.

Moving to Independent Living increases connections to others. Although it is possible to live in an Independent unit and seldom go out of one's apartment, most residents become involved in their new community and participate in classes and activities they enjoy, thus meeting new people and making friends. Communal dining increases contact with others and enhances quality of life.

## Assisted Living

Assisted Living is the next level of care in a Senior Living Complex. Some seniors enter this level of care only when they are no longer able to look after their day-to-day needs in their own homes. For those already in Independent Living, a move to Assisted Living may be necessitated by a fall or a health problem that reduces the senior's ability to continue to care for themselves.

Services include social activities and outings, nutritious meals, housekeeping and maintenance, medication supervision, and personal care.[20] The resident has an apartment, although it may be smaller than those in Independent Living.

As all meals are provided, most apartments have minimal kitchens. Often a microwave, small refrigerator, and sink are the only items. ADA (American Disabilities Act) requirements set the standards for the apartment configuration:

- "Be designed so that all spaces, furnishings, and equipment, including storage units and operable windows, are easily usable by residents in wheelchairs.

- Be equipped with grab bars in all appropriate locations.

- Be free of tripping hazards." [21]

Medical staff is usually not available around the clock, but there is normally a Registered Nurse (RN), Licensed Practical Nurse (LPN) or Vocational Nurse (LVN) in charge.[22] There may be a doctor on call, but residents continue to see their personal doctors. Caregivers are on site 24 hours a day to assist with needed services at all times.

## Memory Care

Seniors enter a Memory Care unit when they can no longer safely live independently or in Assisted Living due to Alzheimer's or some other form of dementia. To be eligible for memory care, a medical diagnosis of dementia is required, as well as the need for around-the-clock supervision.[23] A person entering Memory Care may or may not be handicapped physically. Staffing is determined by state regulations but is at a higher level than Assisted Living. There will normally be a higher ratio of staff during the day and early evening shifts.

Memory Care units provide a safe environment for residents as they are restricted from wandering. The units are locked 24/7, and entry and exit by everyone is carefully controlled.

All activities are designed to enhance the lives of the residents. Music programs are popular as they have a profound effect. Music stimulates areas of the brain not affected by the disease, decreases agitation, and increases communication.[24] Gardening and crafts are other programs that are frequently provided.

## Skilled Nursing (SNF)/Custodial Care

CCRCs usually have a Skilled Nursing Facility/Custodial Care to care for those residents whose needs can no longer be accommodated in Assisted Living. A SNF is usually not considered to be a long-term nursing home but a facility where patients go after discharge from the hospital after surgery or an illness or injury.[25] However, in CCRCs where total life care is needed, this may be combined with Custodial Care.

Custodial care is a popular form of long-term support that helps older adults who need non-medical assistance on a daily or ongoing basis. Those who serve in this capacity don't need a medical background, official training, or certifications. You can receive custodial care in a range of facilities.[26]

Living quarters may be a single or shared room with a bathroom, rather than an apartment. Some shared rooms are divided by a curtain for privacy. A resident may have their own furniture, but space is limited.

### Custodial Care/Short-Term Rehabilitation Facilities

These usually are not part of a senior living complex or the services may be included in an SNF or Custodial Care unit.

# Government Oversight

The Federal government has basic minimum age requirements to live in a designated senior community and all states must follow this rule. In addition, there may be state regulations that apply. Senior communities have a wide range of ages, but the majority of residents enter between the ages of 75 and 84 with the average age of residents being 84[27].

The *Federal Fair Housing Act* exempts Senior Housing complexes if they are recognized by the state or federal government to be designed and operated to meet the needs of the elderly and are restricted to those over the age of 55 or 62.[28] They must still meet ADA requirements and other anti-discrimination statutes.[29]

Because most regulation of senior living communities is determined by the state, there are wide differences in requirements. Independent Living has the fewest requirements in most states, while Assisted Living and higher levels of care have many more. The biggest variant is in the area of staffing, especially the ratio of staff to residents and staff training.[30]

For specific information if you are searching for a community, it is necessary to research the state requirements. This can be especially important if you are considering different states.

Assisted Living and higher-level care facilities are required to have very specific evacuation plans in case of an emergency. Each facility must not only have a plan, but train staff in what their specific roles are during an emergency situation.

As noted previously, Independent Living Communities have fewer regulations because residents are presumed to be capable of handling all their own needs. Independent Living apartment complexes are required to have an evacuation plan, which means clearly identified exits with appropriate signage and fire extinguishers. Beyond this, it is up to the state to determine what other evacuation plans must be in place.

# Summary

Continuing Care Retirement Communities and Month-to-Month Lease Communities have quite different fee structures and operating policies. Your financial situation may determine which type of community you select. Ownership plays a key part and may be a factor in finding the sites that best fit your needs. Deciding whether you are independent enough for Independent Living or if you will be best served in Assisted Living is an important decision.

# How Do You Want to Spend Your Remaining Time?

## Senior Living Services and Activities

Senior Living Communities offer a wide variety of services and activities to enhance the lives of residents. Prepared meals, maintenance, and security are services provided in all senior living communities. These are the very reasons why we leave our homes; to be free of the chores that consume our time and energy and to feel safe in our environment.

# Standard Services

Standard services are the ones you expect to find in all Senior Living Communities. However, there may be differences in how that service is provided because of the level of care.

## Meals

Meals are one of the most important issues, after cost and care, and one which will greatly impact your satisfaction with a given community. For this reason, it's essential to eat *at least* one meal in any community being considered. Far from being just a "free meal," you'll taste the food, experience the atmosphere of the dining room, and observe residents interacting with each other—all of which are important.

## Meals in Independent Living

The number of meals included in your contract and how they are administered varies with the community.

Some communities include one meal, normally dinner, per day as part of your contract. Breakfast and lunch, in addition, may be available for a set cost. Other communities provide two meals per day, usually dinner plus breakfast or lunch. Guest meals are charged to the guest or resident.

If you don't want to deal with preparing any meals yourself, choose a community with a food plan that accommodates this. If you're willing or want to make your own breakfast and/or lunch in your unit, a meal plan with more flexibility may better fit your needs.

Another arrangement is a point system where residents are given a certain number of points per month, specifically for food; alcohol cannot be purchased with the points. These points may be used at any meal and may or may not be spent on guest meals. Unused points may be lost or carried over to the next month. Spending more than your allocated number of points results in a charge on the next month's bill.

Most community dining rooms offer two or three menu choices per meal, including soup or salad and dessert at dinner. This type of menu usually comes with additional "every day" options, such as hamburgers, grilled cheese, etc., for those who do not want the daily specials. Other communities offer a more extensive menu with many choices that change every few months and may include daily specials.

If you have special dietary needs, it's important to find out if the menu options meet or can be adjusted for your requirements. Because Independent Living accommodations are not required to meet diverse dietary needs, this is something you need to know before signing a contract. You can ask to speak to the chef to clarify your needs.

The hours the dining room is open and how residents are seated can vary greatly. Some Independent Living dining rooms are open all day with breakfast, lunch and dinner hours defining the menu available. Others are open several hours for each meal, e.g., breakfast between 7:00 and 10:00, lunch between 11:30 and 1:30 and dinner between 4:00 and 6:00. A less frequent arrangement is when meals are served at set hours, e.g., breakfast at 8:00, lunch at noon, and dinner at 5:00. Take-out meals, available in most communities, are especially useful when you're not feeling well or just want to have a meal in your own unit.

Dining room atmosphere is important. Do people seem to be enjoying their meal, talking and laughing at their tables and speaking to others as they pass by? How friendly and helpful is the wait staff? Is there a bistro, coffee bar, or café for casual between-meals snacks? Does this seem like a place where you'll enjoy spending an hour or more every day?

## Meals in Assisted Living

When you enter Assisted Living, more inclusive meal plans go into effect. Three meals per day are included in the monthly fee, and often, snacks are available at no additional charge. The menu is smaller, with fewer choices. If you're on a medically prescribed diet (diabetes, heart, etc.), check with the facility to see if your personal needs can be met.

Residents are encouraged to have their meals in the dining room, and help is available for those who can't navigate to the dining room by themselves. Tables will usually be for four people to increase the opportunity to socialize.

# Maintenance

One of the advantages of leaving your home and moving to a senior complex is you no longer have to worry about home maintenance. If the sink backs up, an appliance doesn't work, a light burns out on the ceiling, etc., you simply put in a work order, and someone else takes care of the problem.

There is scheduled maintenance for changing filters, washing outside windows, elevator maintenance, fire safety equipment, plumbing, etc. All public areas, e.g., dining room, lobby, laundry areas, elevators, and hallways, are kept in good repair, as are individual units. Before a new resident moves in, the apartment is thoroughly cleaned and made to look like new. Outdoor landscaping and building exteriors are kept neat, clean, and attractive.

# Security

Having a Security Guard on duty, especially at night, is reassuring for residents of senior communities. We all sleep better knowing someone is awake and watching out for us.

24/7 security cameras, providing additional security at all building entrances, are monitored and, if concerns arise, can be reviewed. While the entrance to the lobby is unlocked during the day when a staff member is present, other doors are normally locked. Residents use their apartment keys or a code to enter from parking areas and locked entrances.

# Other Services

In addition to the basic services provided to everyone in a Senior Living facility, there are other services that may be offered. Those listed below are most commonly found.

## Housekeeping

Often, there is yearly cleaning of carpets, windows and vents for both Independent and Assisted Living apartments. Independent Living complexes may provide regular cleaning services for individual units. This can include basic cleaning of kitchens, bathrooms, floors, and dusting. It may include the laundering of sheets and towels. If this service is not provided, you will need to do your basic cleaning or hire someone to do it for you.

Housekeeping of apartments in Assisted Living is part of the service provided for everyone and is more inclusive. It usually includes full laundry service, as washers/dryers are not available for residents.

The list of what is included in housekeeping varies greatly. Ask the sales coordinator what is included and make sure it is stated in your contract.

## Transportation

Many Independent Living residents, and almost all residents in Assisted Living, no longer drive, so transportation is an important service. The vehicles provided vary, but most communities have a bus and/or large van, a smaller van, and perhaps a car or two. These are equipped to be accessible for those with mobility issues.

## Off-site Transportation

Medical visits are the most important use of provided transportation for those living in Independent and Assisted Living. These are scheduled in advance in order to serve all requests in a timely fashion. Forms must be completed with specific information. Do you have a walker or wheelchair? (If you have a scooter, check to see if it can be accommodated.) Do you need transportation round trip? What is the address of your doctor? You will be notified of your pick-up time in advance.

When your appointment is over, the driver will pick you up as soon as possible, but you may need to wait, depending on logistics. It's a good idea to have a bottle of water, a snack and a book or your phone to keep you occupied while you wait.

Often, Independent Living communities offer trips to local shopping areas, banks, and other community locations on a weekly or monthly schedule. If the schedule permits, personal requests for transportation may be accommodated in some communities.

Transportation to local churches, synagogues, and other houses of worship is often available. These may be regularly scheduled for those having large numbers of members living in the Senior Community. However, transportation to other religious sites may be possible if they can be worked into the schedule.

Transportation for activities scheduled by staff is normally provided at no cost. Individual appointments and travel may be included at no charge, depending on availability, or there may be a fee.

## On-site Transportation

Most Senior Living Communities have multiple buildings serving different levels of care. Residents may wish to visit friends or use the services and activities available in other buildings, but many do not have the mobility to do this on their own. For this reason, on-site transportation may be available.

Golf cart type electric vehicles, operated by staff, provide a quick way to get between buildings. These vehicles are not meant to be driven on city streets and have a low speed. Holding between three and seven passengers, the carts transport residents and their mobility devices. Some communities provide this transportation on a regular schedule, some provide it for special programs being held in a specific building, and others provide it upon advance request.

# Gym/ Fitness Centers

## Independent Living

Gyms, or rooms dedicated to exercise and fitness, are part of the Independent Living building design. There may be exercise machines, weights, exercise bars, exercise balls, and chairs for seated exercises. Some have swimming pools for water aerobics and water therapy, as well as independent use.

Exercise classes meet differing levels of physical abilities and focus on core strength, mobility, balance, and flexibility. Yoga, Tai Chi, drumming, and Pilates are also popular. Physical Therapists, Personal Trainers, or on-site staff may teach the classes, or videos may be used in place of an actual instructor. The exercise equipment is available for individuals to use when a class is not in session, but the use of the equipment will be unsupervised.

## Assisted Living

There may be a dedicated exercise room in Assisted Living, but many facilities provide classes in a multi-purpose room. The equipment used includes balls, light weights, bean bags, etc., that can be easily manipulated. There are seldom exercise machines as they may be dangerous if used without supervision.

Seated exercise classes are offered in Assisted Living and there are many adaptations to meet the needs of residents. Classes focus on coordination, balance, strength, and flexibility. Assisted Living swimming pools have devices to help residents enter the water. The pool is not used independently but with supervision. Water aerobics is a popular option when a pool is available.

# Optional Services

## Library

A library is a valued amenity that provides enjoyment for residents. Collections may include large print and audiobooks to meet the needs of those with failing sight, especially in Assisted Living facilities. There may be magnifying devices for those with more extreme sight issues. Daily newspapers are usually available for residents, either in the library or in another common area.

Access is very convenient because the library is located on the premises. Although some are open only at designated hours and have a volunteer checking items in and out, others are open 24/7 on an honor system.

A budget may allow the purchase of magazines, newspapers, and new books, but most of the collection is donated by new residents. As shelf space is limited, a volunteer resident librarian and/or committee decides which donated books are added to the collection and those that are removed as they are no longer being read.

Creating a library philosophy and circulation policy and posting them keeps everyone aware of the goals and purpose of the library.

## Banking

Some Senior complexes have a small branch bank located on the premises. Residents use it as they would any bank; those with accounts at that bank have all the amenities it offers, while those who do not have an account may use the services but with the same additional fees as they would have off-site.

An ATM is another banking service that may be available. Fees are the same as at any bank ATM, but the ease of being able to get cash as needed may outweigh the fees.

## Beauty Shop/Barber

Many complexes offer this valuable service. There may be a salon in each building of a large complex or it may be in a central location in a smaller one. If Assisted Living residents are unable to go to the salon by themselves, the staff will transport them to and from their apartment.

Services provided are hair, nails and sometimes even massage or other spa services. Prices are usually reasonable. Going to the beauty shop/barber helps residents feel better and is a positive experience.

# Bar

## Independent Living

A bar is an amenity that appeals to many residents. It is normally open at set hours, usually late afternoon through dinner and possibly early evening. Wine may be available at dinner. Some communities have a daily "Happy Hour," which may feature special drinks. Others may have a weekly or monthly "Happy Hour" with entertainment. Alcohol charges are added to the monthly bill.

## Assisted Living

Alcohol policies vary greatly in Assisted Living. If the facility has a liquor license, there may be a bar where residents can socialize, or wine may be available at meals.[31] There may be "Happy Hour" activities, with festive alcoholic and non-alcoholic drinks, and New Year's may be celebrated with champagne.

# Pets

Both Independent Living and Assisted Living usually permit residents to have pets, but there may be an additional move-in fee. The rules and regulations vary, so it's important to know if your pet qualifies. Size is often the primary guideline for acceptance. Pets provide companionship and decrease feelings of being alone. They're also a good icebreaker when meeting new people. People who bring their pets with them when they move tend to feel at home more quickly.

There may be dog-walking social groups or activities planned for those with dogs. There may be pet walkers who can take your dog for longer walks if you are unable to do so.

If you have a dog, check out the pet area and where you can go for walks. You may want to get an apartment conveniently located so you don't have to walk far in inclement weather. If there is a fenced dog yard, are there chairs where you can sit? Is the area clean? Are there bags and a closed trash can available?

Cats are a little easier than dogs. If you have a cat, look at apartments with an eye to where you will put the litter box. Do the windows have ledges where your cat can sit and look out?

It's important to have plans in place for who will care for your pet if you suddenly must go to the hospital or become incapacitated and unable to care for them.

## Activities

Being free of the minutia of daily living makes our lives much easier, and we now have hours of free time at our disposal. Perhaps for the first time since we were very young, there may be no demands on us, and we can pursue our lives as we want.

There is time to explore hobbies and interests we didn't have enough time for previously, or we can find new interests we never knew we had. Activities include those regularly scheduled and special events and/or speakers and programs.

A monthly calendar provides information about every activity taking place during the month. There will be a diverse array of options to entice people to take part in activities that appeal to them.

## Regularly Scheduled Classes and Activities

Many classes recur weekly, and a few may be offered daily. Exercise classes help residents keep fit and lessen the chances of falling. Arts and crafts classes encourage creativity, while topical issues discussion groups keep our brains sharp.

Bingo, Corn Hole, Trivia and other games are popular in many communities and may be offered weekly. While some games, like Bridge, demand some level of competence to join, most only require you to show up and participate. Other activities may include in-house movies, gardening, and cooking classes.

Suggestions for activities not currently on the schedule can be made to the Activities Director. They are often willing to try new options, and if there is enough response, an activity will be added to the ongoing calendar.

## Outings

Independent Living communities usually offer a number of outings for residents each month. These may include concerts, plays, festivals, and community events, as well as museums and local places of interest. All outings include the necessary transportation. The staff may purchase tickets, but residents pay individually, usually on their monthly bill. Some advantages of going as part of a group are that there may be discounts, and you don't have to walk a long way from the parking lot or stand in long lines to purchase tickets.

Trips to restaurants are especially enjoyed by many residents. The restaurants vary in menu, cost, and location to provide variety and interest. Reservations are made by the Activities Department, and each resident pays for their own meal. Residents sit together, providing an opportunity to get to know each other better.

## Performances and Programs

The number and type of programs provided vary greatly by level of care. Music performances are the most universal. "The positive effects [of music] include improved mood, cognition, physical health, QOL [Quality of Life] and well-being, spirituality, sleep, increased socialization, and communication. There is also evidence of reduced depression, anxiety, stress, agitation and behavior problems, as well as fewer medical interventions. Music has an integral part in elder care, and studies continue to show its relevance.[32]

Independent Living residents are often offered a wide array of performances and lectures. Some are purely for entertainment, such as singing and dancing groups, comedians, or travel shows. Others stimulate thinking, such as a *League of Women Voters* discussion of ballot issues, instructions on what to do if you fall, or a lecture about the Apollo space missions.

## Resident Councils and Committees

Many Independent Living and some Assisted Living communities have a Resident Council, or Association made up of volunteers elected by residents. Officers may be a President, Vice President, and Secretary with other officers included as necessary. The Council communicates with management to enhance understanding, learn new information, and resolve issues.

41

In addition, there may be volunteer resident committees based on specific areas of interest to the residents. These meet regularly to discuss specific concerns and suggestions of residents and report back to the community through regularly scheduled meetings, minutes, and newsletters. They may also welcome new residents and help them make the transition to their new home.

## Additional Services

There are many additional services that may be offered. No individual site will have all of them, but you may look for those that are of special interest to you, such as a chapel, tennis or pickleball courts, a small on-site mart for purchasing incidentals, a greenhouse, or putting greens (some communities are even adjacent to a golf course). Helping you stay healthy, a site may schedule visits from a podiatrist, dentist, or hearing aid tune-up specialist. A physical therapist may be available for individual appointments. Some of these may be at no cost, or there may be a fee attached.

Other services you may appreciate are a concierge, package delivery and/ or mailing, secure shredder, visitor screening, resale shops for residents, technology assistance, and personal safety devices. If there's something you especially want or need, discuss its availability with your sales representative.

# Summary

Services and activities will vary from site to site, but all communities include some basic services: meals, transportation, security, and maintenance. Additional services may include housekeeping, a fitness center, a library, banking, a beauty shop/barber, a bar, and pets.

Activities include a wide variety of scheduled classes and games, outings, performances and programs. There may be a resident council/association and committees to coordinate resident issues and concerns with management.

# Going on a Treasure Hunt

## Searching For Your New Home

Having read Chapters One—Three, you understand the basics of senior living and are preparing for a move to a senior living complex. When you're ready to start actively searching, the first step is compiling a list of communities to visit. Searching only for communities that meet your criteria will save time and energy.

# Narrowing the Field

### Finances

Your first decision is what type community fits your needs and budget. Is a CCRC or a month-to-month lease the best choice for you? If you want a CCRC, what is the maximum you are willing and able to pay for the buy-in? In either case, how much can you afford to pay for the monthly rent, knowing there are likely to be yearly increases for inflation?

Do you qualify for a government or military supported community? If so, how much of your income will you be expected to pay? Is there enough left in your monthly income for other living expenses?

### Independent or Assisted Living

Next, you need to determine whether you belong in Independent Living or Assisted Living. How is your overall health? If you have concerns about whether you're physically and mentally fit enough for Independent Living, discuss your concerns with your doctor.

This decision may be a result of how long you've waited to move from your home. If every day living has become much too difficult, you may want to move directly to Assisted Living. If you are moving to make life easier and less stressful and can easily navigate living on your own, Independent Living will meet your needs.

Sometimes, future residents assess themselves as being able to live independently only to discover they belong in Assisted Living. The realization of a poor fit may be apparent almost immediately, or it may take several months. However, not only is the process of moving, in and of itself, very stressful but uprooting again within a short period of time, can be overwhelming.

There may be additional fees related to another move as well as the cost of physically moving the contents of your apartment. It's best to move to the appropriate facility when you make your initial move.

## Family and Community

Being near family, if possible, is a primary consideration for many elders. If you have family nearby, there may be no question; you want to remain in the same general vicinity where you currently live. If your family is far-flung, you may want to consider moving to a community closer to one of them. Positive family ties enhance life in a senior community through shared meals, holidays, and activities. Relatives may also be called on in a crisis. Before moving to be closer to a relative, however, consider the following questions:

- How close are you to this relative?

- How available is the relative to provide help when necessary?

- How much time does the relative have to spend with you?

- Has the relative expressed a desire to have you move close to them?

- Is the relative willing to take on a support role for you?

- Is this relative located where other family members can easily visit?

If you are planning to move away from the area where you presently live, be sure you know and understand the greater community where you'll be moving. Even though we live in the same country, lifestyles, beliefs, and customs vary greatly, and you want your new community to be a good fit. You don't want to relocate half-way across the country, or even across your state or city, and discover you don't have much in common with those in your new community.

## Defining Your Needs

To make your site visit as useful as possible, some specifics will help the sales team narrow your search. Tell them whether you want an apartment or cottage and the size you prefer: studio, one-bedroom, two-bedroom, one bathroom or two. If you aren't sure what you want, ask to see samples of all you're considering. Let them know if you want to move in fairly quickly. If there are amenities you desire, be sure to ask about them.

The *Community Information Work Sheet* at the end of this chapter, provides a guideline of what to look for during your visit and provides you with a way to remember the details about each individual site.

# Selecting Potential Sites

## Senior Referral Services

There are a number of referral services that will find the senior communities that best meet your identified needs. These referral services can be located on-line by searching for "senior living referral agencies." You will be asked a series of questions regarding health, location, finances, etc. The agency will then send you a list of potential sources and you personally contact these communities for visits. There is no fee to you for this service. If you select a community from the list, the agency receives a finder's fee from the site you selected.

This service is especially helpful if you plan to move a distance away from your current home. It can narrow your search and save time by selecting only the communities that appear to be the best fits. It can also be helpful if you feel overwhelmed by the number of options available in your area.

## Compile Your Own List of Sites

If you want to make your own list of potential communities, you may need to do a bit of research. If you live in a small community, your options may be limited and location may be your deciding factor. However, expanding your search within a reasonable radius may permit you to find a better fit.

Those living in metropolitan areas have numerous options, but not all will be a good match. The larger the city, the more options available and narrowing the number of sites to visit is essential. For instance, San Diego has 156 identified communities and *US Health*

*News* reports 420 communities are available in Chicago! Begin your search within a small radius, keeping in mind travel time for family. Using the criteria you compiled previously, choose those that appear to fit best by reviewing their web sites.

You may be aware of some communities because you have friends living there; you may even have visited. If your impression is good, put them on your list to visit; if you have concerns, don't include them. Expand your search area as necessary, always keeping in mind the distance from family. With your list of plausible sites, you are ready to make appointments to visit in person.

## On-Site Visits

An on-site visit, before signing a contract, is essential. If you're not personally able to tour the community, a tour by a family member or friend is the next best option. Video tours may be available, but they do not give the more complete picture you find through a personal visit. There are many nuances to what will be a good fit and what will not, and the best way to know for sure is to visit in person.

Your first step is to make appointments to visit those communities that most appeal to you from the research you've done. Unless you're visiting an area from out of town, don't schedule more than one site visit per day and, if possible, allow at least a couple of days between visits. If you have even more time before you feel you want to move, you can schedule your visits further apart. This gives you time to think about each site after the visit and consider how well you think it will fit your needs.

If you live in a city and have many options, check out *at least* four different communities. If you are not pressed for time, go to as many as look feasible. The more sites you visit, the better you can choose the one that is best for you.

## Schedule Your Visit

Choose a time for your visit when residents are likely to be active; late morning is ideal. Be sure your visit includes a meal to help you get a sense of the dining experience you'll have every day. Allow plenty of time so you won't feel rushed.

## Initial Visit

Use your *Community Information Work Sheet* *(see end of this chapter)* to make sure you are shown all areas important to you. Ask lots of questions. The sales team's objective is to sign you up and to do this they will paint the best picture possible. While you're walking the halls, be aware of what's going on. Are residents out and about? What are they doing? Stop and talk to residents when possible.

In addition to the glossy sales brochures you'll be given, ask for copies of all literature available for residents; monthly calendars, newsletters, committee reports, minutes of meetings, etc.

Continue visiting possible communities until you have a list of two—four that you feel will meet your needs.

## Second Visits

You've visited the senior communities you identified as possible future homes. For whatever reason, you wrote off some immediately; you knew they weren't where you want to spend your remaining years. For the ones you are still considering, you have files with information on each of the sites.

When you've identified the communities, you think will be appropriate for you, it's time to go back for a second visit. Never make your decision based on a single visit. If you're from out of town and have limited time, it's still very important to go back for a second visit to learn more before you commit.

Limit your second visits to no more than three of four communities, those you believe are the best fit for you. Again, make appointments; preferably at a different time than your first visit. If you had lunch on your first visit, dinner time gives you an opportunity to see public areas in a different light, observe how residents are interacting, and sample another meal.

Some Independent Living communities have apartments where you can spend a few days actually experiencing life as it might be as a resident. Although this will not be the same as living there, you will gain a better idea if this is a fit for you.

Bringing family members, or a friend, along on your second visit is a good idea. They know you well and may ask questions you haven't thought about. They also may have a sense of how you might fit into the community. The decision is yours, but the more input you have, the better.

Bring a list of questions you thought of after your initial visit. When you were starting your search, you may have been overwhelmed by everything you saw. There are almost sure to be questions about things you didn't think of or forgot to ask. Other questions may have come up since your initial visit.

During this second visit, try to picture yourself living there. Can you visualize how it would be to experience this scenario from the inside instead of from the outside looking in? Talk to as many residents as possible. Ask them why they like living there. Are they enthusiastic? The more residents you talk to, the better picture you will build in your mind.

Ask if there are any discounts being offered. Some communities offer discounts for veterans or there may be a discount if you are a member of the sponsoring agency that owns the community. Sometimes there may be a special offer that reduces the rent or the move-in costs.

Ask to see all currently available apartments in your defined configuration (one or two bedrooms, etc.) If there is one you especially like, and you feel ready to commit, ask to reserve it. You may be able to have it held for a few days at no cost or you may need to pay a refundable, or partially refundable, deposit. You are not ready to sign a contract at this stage, no matter how sure you are so don't rush the process.

If, after two visits, you're still wavering about which community to choose, go back for a third visit. Don't feel like you're imposing on anyone by doing this. It's the job of the sales staff to recruit new residents and they cheerfully will meet with you as many times as necessary to get you to commit.

## Other Opportunities for Gathering Information

Some communities have monthly social events for prospective residents. Or, there may be a celebration for a new facility or an anniversary, to which the general public is invited. If you're invited to one of these, be sure to go. Although it will not be a realistic view of life in that community, it's an opportunity to meet some residents and talk on an informal basis. You will also meet additional staff members. By mingling, you learn more about what the community is like. Be aware, however, this is an opportunity to "sell" the public on the community's image and is probably not representative of the day-to-day life that takes place there.

Talk to your friends and family about the communities you are considering. They may know residents or have knowledge that may be helpful. If their comments raise questions for you, write them down to address later.

# Signing the Contract

## Prior to Signing

Before you sign on the dotted line, you need to decide on the specific apartment you want and your move-in date. Your choice is limited to apartments currently vacant. If none of these are what you want, you may go on a waiting list to be notified when the exact type of apartment you want becomes available.

If the apartment you want has already been refurbished, your move-in date can be negotiated with staff. If the apartment recently became available, you may need to wait for renovations to be completed. Regardless, when you sign your contract, you commit to a specific move-in date.

The contract specifies the apartment and the date you'll take possession. You don't need to physically occupy the apartment on the designated date, but your monthly rent will begin then. Some seniors, although they are not ready to move for a few weeks, or even months, want the security of having a specific apartment available when they're ready and they're willing to pay for that.

Usually there are only a few apartment configurations available in a single building; all studios or two bedroom/ two bath apartments will be identical or nearly so. The difference is primarily in view and placement of the apartment within the building. For some, this isn't as important as being able to move in immediately; for others, it's worth waiting to get an apartment that meets their own criteria. And, whether you physically move in immediately, or days or months later; when your move-in date arrives, you are entitled to use all amenities and services.

## Signing the Contract

When you decide to enter a senior living community, you'll sign a contract. There are four types of contracts, CCRC contracts are normally Type A, B, or C while month to month rental contracts usually fall into Type D.

- Type A Contracts are the most expensive as all health care is prepaid. You will be cared for and housed at no, or minimal, additional cost for all levels of care for the remainder of your life.

- Type B Contracts are a modified life care contract and include entrance and service fees and partial prepayment for extended levels of health service. The monthly fee may increase as the level of care increases and the entire cost of the new level of care may not be paid.

- Type C Contracts require fees for service. Although they are less in initial buy-in, as higher levels of service are needed, the resident must pay these costs out of pocket.

- Type D Contracts are rental (month-to-month) contracts and are not often available in a CCRC. There is no buy-in fee and all services are on a pay-as-you-go basis.[33]

If you've selected a community with a Type A, B, or C contract, it may include a refund option. "Refund options for CCRCs may range from no refund after an initial adjustment period, a refund amount that declines over time, or a stated percentage refund. CCRC contracts with attractive refund provisions must require entry fee payments that are significantly higher than non-refundable contracts." [34]

If you are unsure of the type of contract you are signing, ask your marketing coordinator. Get a copy of the contract and take it home so you can study and understand it. Mark any areas where you have questions. The contract may be long and written in legalese making it difficult to understand, but the details are important.

There may be lists of things like candles, guns, etc. that residents are not permitted to have. If, for any reason, you want to have something on the forbidden list, discuss it with the appropriate staff member. If you reach an agreement that you may have it, put it into writing in the contract. For example, if you have an antique gun in a display case, you may be given an exemption for it. If so, write it into the contract.

There may be a list of reasons why you may be asked to leave the facility. Be sure you understand exactly what these are. If you have any concerns about the contract or aspects you don't understand, you may want to check with an attorney before signing.

If rent increases are not specified in the contract, ask what they have been in the past and what the maximum increase is per year. Again, put this into the contract.

All promises made by the marketing staff should be put into writing. If you have been given a discount for any reason, make sure it is clearly stated in the contract. If you want to move in immediately, but the apartment you want is currently not available, you may want to move into a different apartment until one becomes available. Put the agreement in writing that you will be given priority and won't be charged additional fees.

After you've negotiated any concerns and feel the contract is acceptable, sign it and get a copy for your files. In most cases, you'll never need it, but if a dispute should arise, you'll have a copy of the official contract to verify your case.

## Summary

Finding a senior community that is the best fit for you is important. Your first step is defining what you want. This includes looking at your finances and deciding whether you want a CCRC or a month-to-month contract. You'll also need to determine whether you belong in Independent Living or Assisted Living. Family and community need to be considered as well as what you require in the number of bedrooms and bathrooms.

You can find potential sites by using a referral service or devising your own list. On-site visits narrow your options and help you decide. Finally, you will want to make sure you understand the contract and that any added agreements are in writing and signed.

# Community Information
## Work Sheet

Name _____

Phone Number _____

Contact Name And Number _____

| OWNER | Corporate | Religious | Other |
|---|---|---|---|

## GENERAL

| | | | |
|---|---|---|---|
| **Grounds** | Walkways | Green areas | Sitting areas |
| **Entry/ Lobby** | | Welcoming | Convenient |
| **Halls** | Attractive | Clean | Well-lit |
| **Elevator(s)** | | Convenient | Clean |
| **Gym/ Exercise Room** | | Yes | No |
| **Arts & Crafts Room** | | Yes | No |
| **Beauty/ Barber Shop** | | Yes | No |
| **Game Room** | | Yes | No |
| **Theater** | | Yes | No |
| **Library** | | Yes | No |
| **Bar** | | Yes | No |
| **Parking for Residents** | Covered | Outdoor | Cost _____ |
| **Parking for Guests** | | Convenient | Abundant |
| **Electric Car Charging Stations** | | Yes | No |

| Friendliness of Residents | Very | | Somewhat | Unknown |
|---|---|---|---|---|
| Transportation | No Cost | | Minimal Cost | Other |
| Wi-Fi, Cable | Included | N/C | Group Rate | Not Included |

## DINING

| | | | |
|---|---|---|---|
| **Quality of Food** | Excellent | Good | Poor |
| **Diversity of Menu** | Excellent | Good | Poor |
| **Ambiance of Dining Room** | Excellent | Good | Poor |
| **Acoustics** | Excellent | Good | Poor |
| **Meal Plan** | Meals included in rent | | |

Cost for meals not included

_____

## ACTIVITIES

**How many of activities on monthly calendar are of interest to you?**

_____

## APARTMENT/ COTTAGE

| | | | | |
|---|---|---|---|---|
| **Size of unit** | Studio | 1 Bedroom | 2 Bedroom | Other |
| **Monthly Rent** | $_____ | | | |
| **Bedroom(s)** | Size_____ | | | |
| **Closets** | Large | | Small | |
| **Living Room** | Size _____ | | | |
| **Dining Area** | Size _____ | | | |
| **Balcony/ Patio** | Yes | | No | |

| **Kitchen Appliances** | Refrigerator | Stove | Microwave | Dishwasher | Disposal |
|---|---|---|---|---|---|

| **Cabinets Accessibility** | | Good | | Difficult | |
|---|---|---|---|---|---|

| **Cabinets Capacity** | Good | Satisfactory | | Poor | |
|---|---|---|---|---|---|

| **Bathrooms** | 1 full | 2 full | 1 ½ | | Other |
|---|---|---|---|---|---|

| **Walk-in shower** | Yes | No | | | |
|---|---|---|---|---|---|

**Handicap toilet**     Yes     No

**Grab Bars**     Yes     No

**Heating/AC**     In Unit     Central

**Washer/ Dryer**     In Unit     Shared     Central Facility     N/A

**Storage**     Plentiful     Adequate     Lacking

**Lighting**     Good     Satisfactory     Poor

**Sufficient Electrical Outlets**     Yes     No

**Cleaning**     Yes     No

**View**     Excellent     Satisfactory     Disappointing

**Resident Association**     Yes     No

**Pets Allowed**     Yes     No     Fee _____

**Designated Pet Area**     Yes     No

## Other (Add anything you like or need):

# Too Much Stuff!

## Downsizing

Most of us have more household goods and personal items than we're able to take with us when we move to a senior living complex. Having lived in the same home for 30, 40, or more years, we may have accumulated "stuff" we don't even remember we have. But no matter how long you've lived in your home, you must decide what will go with you and what you'll need to dispose of. Where to begin?

You can hire a professional downsizing expert, also known as a Senior Mover, to help you select what to keep for your new life and what to do with all that remains. The expert works with you, taking into consideration your personal lifestyle as well as the space you'll have available. *If you are hiring a professional who will facilitate your downsizing and move, you can skip to the next chapter.*

For those of you who are going to handle downsizing yourselves, the remainder of this chapter will help you decide what to move and how to get rid of what is left.

# What to Take

## Furniture

Having a limited amount of space in your new apartment, you'll want to carefully choose the furniture to take. Before you begin to make decisions, you need a floor plan for each room in your new home.

Many communities have floor plans with dimensions available on their website, or you can ask if a print copy is available. If not, you can draw each room of your floor plan to approximate size on graph paper. Be sure to include doors (including closets and built-in cabinet doors).

Wall plugs and TV/Wi-Fi connections should be noted. You may need to return for another visit to visually locate them as this impacts your furniture placement. Where is the thermostat? You'll need clear access to this.

When you're deciding what furniture to put in each room, consider pieces that can serve more than one purpose. For example, a dining table may fold up to become an occasional table, dining room chairs may serve as living room chairs, or a cedar chest may serve as a coffee table. Be creative to make the best use of your beloved items.

There are several ways to develop a furniture placement plan depending on the way you process information. You may want to make copies of the blank floor plan for backup.

- Option #1: Cut a piece of paper to the appropriate dimensions of each piece of furniture. Move the furniture into various configurations to see what will work best.

- Option #2: Sketch in the furniture, adding up the total number of feet to be sure it fits. Use a pencil so you can make changes as needed.

- Intuitively, visualize where each item will go and write the name of the piece of furniture on the floor plan.

Be sure all lamps are close to an electrical outlet, and your TV and computer are near the necessary connections.

# Kitchen

If you're moving to Assisted Living, check with the facility for specifics of what small appliances are permitted. As all meals are provided, your kitchen needs are minimal. There are normally no restrictions for Independent Living.

Think about how you'll use your new kitchen. You're moving to a senior complex that provides at least some meals, so how much cooking will you do? You may continue to cook some meals or even have family and friends come to your apartment for meals. If your joy in moving to a senior complex is never having to cook a meal again, at the very least, you'll still warm up leftovers or enjoy a dish of ice cream.

Even if you think you won't cook at all, some basic kitchen items are essential. Plates, cereal/soup bowls, cups, flatware, an assortment of glasses, and a few serving dishes for snacks are needed by almost everyone. Include some storage containers, a mixing bowl or two, a few pots and pans, a coffee pot, and a toaster. You may want to include a countertop microwave, toaster oven, or air fryer. A few kitchen tools, such as a can opener, corkscrew, large spoon, spatula, and jar opener/gripper, will make life easier.

For those who plan to do more cooking, you know which kitchen items you use often and cannot live without. However, remember space may be limited and you need to carefully weigh the value of the small appliances you think you'll use. A crock pot and a blender may be tools you'll use frequently. Beyond that, decide if there are other small appliances you need and want. Will you really use the bread mixer? The waffle iron? The ice cream churn? If so, take them; if not, don't use precious space for something you'll never use.

For some of us, our sterling silver and china are our pride and joy. You may want to take yours with you if you plan to entertain. If not, find a new home where they'll be appreciated. If your children or family members are interested, pass them on now. Unfortunately, many of our children don't want china and silverware as their lifestyle doesn't include formal dining. If no one wants them, consider using them for your everyday set or selling them. (Unfortunately, there isn't a big market for china and the work of trying to sell your dishes may be more difficult than it's worth.)

The amount of shelf and counter space in your new kitchen determines how much you can take with you. When figuring out the amount of shelving available, make sure you only count the shelves you can easily reach; some apartments have shelving too high for most seniors to reach without a step stool, and step stools are not recommended.

## Art, Décor, and Mirrors

To make your new apartment feel like home, you'll want to take your favorite pictures and art objects. Look carefully at what you have. If you love it, take it. Don't worry about where it will be placed. It may end up in a totally different location in your new home, but being surrounded by meaningful décor is important. And, if you later decide there is no place in your new home for a picture or mirror, you can always dispose of it then.

## Photographs and Memorabilia

Only take those photos and memorabilia you plan to display or look at frequently. Much of what you have stored away you haven't looked at in years and, if you stayed where you are currently, would not look at in the future.

## Books and Media

Those of us who are readers have probably collected a lot of books over the years. Even though we may never re-read them, we like feeling we can. They're like friends. However, shelf space will probably be limited in your apartment, so you must take only those books you can't bear to part with. If you have the player and a few favorite CDs, DVDs, etc., take them, but only a few. Chances are you won't play them as much as you think you will.

# Disposing of What You Don't Take

This isn't an easy part of downsizing If you're like most of us, there will be some (or maybe a lot!) of furniture and other large and small items you won't be moving to your new home. What do you do with all of this?

## Furniture

- **Give items to family members and/or friends.**

There may be people in your family or among your friends who would like and appreciate some of the furniture and other items you are unable to use. Those who are just starting their adult lives on their own may be happy to add to their meager amount of furniture. Others may want something that has been in the family and has keepsake value for them.

- **Have an estate sale.**

There are companies that arrange and conduct sales of everything you're not taking with you. If you have many items, the sale may take place in your home, or if you have a smaller amount, your things may be combined with others for a bigger sale elsewhere or online. If you're ambitious and have the energy, you can even have your own estate sale. (You'll still have to deal with what doesn't sell if you do it yourself.)

- **Donate to charity.**

There are numerous charities that will take your unneeded items. Some are designated to help specific populations such as the homeless who are being housed, Veterans, or *Habitat for Humanity*. Others, like *Salvation Army, Goodwill, etc.,* sell donated items and use the money to support those who need it. You may want to arrange for a charity pick-up a month or more in advance as they may be limited in pick-up times, so don't wait to call until the last minute.

- **Arrange to leave for the new owner of your house.**

The buyer of your home may appreciate some of the furniture you cannot take, especially if they're upsizing. Have your realtor inquire if the new owner is interested.

- **Junk disposal.**

A reputable junk disposal company will take everything you are getting rid of. They'll later go through what they collect, separate out what can be donated or recycled, and send what remains to the landfill. You'll have to pay for this service.

- **Storage**

You may be undecided about whether you'll need or be able to use some of your furniture and other objects in your new apartment. Renting a storage locker for a short while gives you the flexibility to keep these things and decide what to do with them when you're actually living in your new home. Renting a storage locker can make the move less stressful because you can keep things you're unsure about. You can check with your community to see if they have available storage.

The caveat here is to make a promise to yourself to only put things in storage that you **really** may want to use. Plan to keep the storage locker for no more than six months. After that, if you haven't needed or wanted something in the locker, keeping it longer is just eating up money, adding stress, and keeping you from totally freeing yourself for your new life.

## Photos and Memorabilia

Getting rid of our personal mementos is hard, especially when we've stored boxes and boxes of things that are meaningful to us. Parting with them is difficult, but *something must be done* with them. There are really only two options for those you won't be taking with you.

- **Give them to their rightful owner.**

Do they belong to someone else? Maybe your children have stored *their* memorabilia in your home. You may have things you saved from your children's childhoods (baby books, pictures and crafts they made, report cards, etc.) Ask your children to claim any of these they want.

You may have memorabilia from your family of origin. See if any of your relatives are interested in having them.

- **Throw them out.**

This is very hard to do, but at some point, someone will throw them out. If you're not going to look at them again, enjoy the experience of reliving the memories and then dispose them in the trash or recycle bin.

## Books and Media

You may have a lot of books and media items that you've decided not to take with you to your new home. What do you do with them?

- **Sell them.**

If you have collectors' books or books with esoteric subjects, you may want to sell them. If this collection is quite large and valuable, hiring an appraiser may be worthwhile. Otherwise, there are quite a few online platforms you can consider.

However, selling them yourself is a time-consuming process and not something to be started while you're in the midst of transitioning to senior living. Either take these books with you in specially marked boxes or store them in a secure, temperature-controlled location, until you're ready to deal with them.

Selling media items is much more difficult and may not be worth the time and effort it takes.

- **Give them to friends and/or colleagues.**

You probably have family and friends who would love to have some of your books and/or media. Invite them over to choose what they might like. If you have up-to-date books relating to your profession, your colleagues may appreciate receiving them.

- **Give them to the library at your new building.**

Libraries in senior living communities depend primarily on donated books from new residents for much of their collection. But space in these libraries is usually limited, so select books you believe will be of interest to the community as a whole and that are in good condition. Fiction, popular non-fiction, large print, and books-on-tape are often welcomed. Other media will probably not be wanted.

- **Give them to your neighborhood library's *Friends of the Library.***

Many *Library Friends* sponsor book sales to raise money to help their local library. This money is used to support the library and its programs. However, before donating, check to make sure your local library wants books and/or media. If they do, ask for their guidelines. If you do donate, make sure all items are in good condition and are of general interest.

- **Repurpose them.**

Although you won't want to repurpose them now, you may want to save some of your old books and media for projects when you're resettled. Many creative options can be found online for ways to make use of old books and media items.

- **Put them in the recycle or trash bin.**

Your college texts, other old and/or worn-out books will not be of interest to anyone; put them in the recycle bin. Old media items may be recycled, but usually not in your curbside collection, so, hard as it is, put them in the trash bin.

## Summary

Downsizing is the most emotional part of the physical move. Although there is still more work to be done before you're finally settled, you'll be looking forward instead of back. Each item you let go of had some emotion tied to it. Even a piece of furniture you never really liked may have had a memory attached.

It's hard to say goodbye to all the things that evoke your past, but you'll feel a little lighter when you're finished. You no longer have that nagging feeling in the back of your mind that you really need to clean out the attic or that storage cabinet. You've done it!

# A Journey of Change: from Here to There

## Moving

As a senior, you've moved at least several times in your life and are familiar with the process. However, it may have been many years since you've moved, and this move may be a little different, especially if you're moving to a senior rental community. If you're moving to a CCRC, your move may be more like what you've experienced in the past.

When you own your house, you must decide whether to keep it, sell it, or rent it. If you plan to sell, will it be before you move or after? If you're living in a rental apartment, give your agreed-upon notice, usually 30 days or on termination of your lease, and you're ready to move. If you currently rent, skip ahead in this chapter to "Step Two, Finding a Moving Company."

# Step One: What to Do with Your Current Home

## Sell before Moving

Selling a house is a fluid process, and there is no way to predict how long it will take to complete the deal. Hopefully your house will sell in a timely manner with no escrow problems, but it doesn't hurt to be thinking of what you'll do in case it sells faster or takes longer than anticipated.

- *Advantages of Selling before Moving*
  - o   Houses sell better when they're furnished and look lived in.

o You'll have your home equity to use for a buy-in for a CCRC, move-in fees and expenses, and/or investments for your future needs.

o If you're still making payments on your house, they will stop once the house is sold.

o You move ahead with your new life with no strings attached to the past.

- *Disadvantages of Selling before Moving*

    o A tight timeline may increase the stress of your move.

    o Your house may sell faster than anticipated, and your new home may not be ready for you. In this case, you probably have two options:

        ▪ You may negotiate delaying your move-out date or rent your house back from the new owner for a month or two.

        ▪ You may need to put everything you plan to take to your new home into storage and dispose of the rest. You'll also need to find a place to live until you can complete your move.

## Keep It or Sell after Moving

You may want more time to decide what to do with your house or not want the stress of selling your house while moving. With this option, you can concentrate on the moving process. When you've moved out, your house will be empty, or at least partially empty.

- *Advantages*

  - You're completely flexible and can move when your new home is ready.

  - You don't need a storage unit; everything you don't move is still available.

  - If the real estate market is unfavorable, you can wait to sell until it becomes more favorable.

  - You may begin by having only essentials and large items moved and add smaller pieces of furniture, pictures, knick-knacks, etc., as you decide what you want.

  - You don't have to sever your contact with the past at the same time you're moving to a new life. You can revisit your house whenever you like.

- *Disadvantages*

  - You won't have your home equity to use as a down payment for a CCRC, move-in expenses, or moving costs.

  - You may not make as much effort to wholeheartedly create a new life for yourself when you know you can always return to your house.

  - You have the expense of keeping up a house where no one lives.

  - You may need to pay for services you previously did yourself, e.g., yard care, snow removal, etc.

  - You may need to hire a security company or install additional security hardware, as no one will be living in the house.

o   If you no longer drive, going back and forth between your new home and old house becomes a logistical problem. If you do drive, you may go back and forth more frequently than necessary.

## Rent It

Renting can be a compromise between keeping your house and selling it.

- *Advantages:*

  o   You receive a relatively steady income from the monthly rent.

  o   You can time your move for when you're ready, and your new residence becomes available.

- *Disadvantages:*

  o   You won't get the equity from your house to pay for a CCRC down payment, moving costs, or to invest for your future needs.

  o   You'll need to hire a property management company to vet potential renters, collect rents, and handle maintenance issues.

  o   You'll pay taxes on your income from the rent as well as continue to pay property taxes.

  o   You're still emotionally tied to the house.

  o   You may have to spend some money to prepare the house for rental.

## Bridge Loans

If your house doesn't sell before you're ready to move or if you want to wait to sell, a bridge loan — also referred to as a gap loan or a swing loan — "is a short-term loan that typically helps with financing when moving from one house to another. Bridge loans are often secured by your current home, but some allow for other types of assets." [35]

# Step Two: Choosing a Moving Company and Services

Having decided what to do with your house, you're ready to plan your move. The community where you're moving may have a list of moving companies they recommend. Get quotes from one or two of these, as well as from at least one national and one local company, not on the list, to get an idea of what the services and costs will be.

If you're moving a long distance, you may want to investigate using portable storage containers instead of hiring a moving company. Containers are brought to your house, and over a specific time period, usually 30 days, you pack the container yourself or hire someone to do this job. When you're finished, you contact the company, and they move the container to your new home where you, or someone you hire, unloads it and the company takes the container away when it's empty. The container company may also store your container (for an additional fee) until you're ready for it.

A full-service moving company usually offers additional assistance beyond actually moving your household goods. The most common are packing and unpacking.

# Packing

You may want to pay the moving company to pack everything for you, or you may want to pack yourself. You may also choose to have the movers pack some things while you do the rest.

- *Advantages of Moving Company Packing:*

    o You don't have to do the hard work of packing.

    o All necessary boxes, crates, packing materials, etc., are provided.

    o Movers are experienced in packing and know how best to wrap and pack different items for safe transit.

    o Movers do all the packing in hours, not days or weeks.

    o You have the use of everything in your house until the last day or so before the move.

- *Disadvantages of Moving Company Packing:*

    o The moving company will tell you when the packers will be at your house. You may not have a say in when that will be.

    o *Everything* in the house will be packed, including trash in wastebaskets and dirty dishes, unless you have clearly marked items not to be packed. You'll need to complete the work of downsizing before the packers arrive.

    o If you're going to do the unpacking, things may not be labeled as you would label them.

o  When everything is packed, unless you've planned ahead for meals (food, dishes, and utensils), you'll need to have take-out or go out for meals until after your move.

- *Advantages of Packing Yourself:*

  o  You have time to sort through and decide what you actually want to take as you pack.

  o  You can pack a last box or two with things you'll want to use immediately and mark them appropriately.

  o  You can mark boxes with designations other than "kitchen," "living room," etc.

  o  It saves money.

- *Disadvantages of Packing Yourself:*

  o  You must buy or collect the boxes and packing materials needed.

  o  It takes a lot of time to pack and label boxes.

  o  Dishes, glasses and other breakables must be wrapped individually with enough packing or bubble wrap to protect them. A box with dividers is helpful for safely packing glassware, but they still need to be wrapped.

  o  You must be careful not to pack things you may need to use before your move.

You may want to do most of the packing and have the moving company pack some unwieldy or fragile items like large pictures and mirrors, china, heirlooms and clothes.

If you're going to be unpacking yourself, one or two boxes should be designated "**ESSENTIAL**." You want items you'll need for the first few days in your new home in this box. Included should be:

- Pillows, sheets and blankets

- Set of towels

- Bathroom necessities

- Coffee pot and ground coffee, instant coffee, or tea bags

- Some disposable plates, cups, silverware and paper towels

- Bottle of wine (Optional)

- Anything else you know for sure you'll need or want at first.

You'll probably have some food and staples left in your refrigerator even though you were using up what you could. If you're moving into your new home in the next day or so, pack an ice chest with the leftovers. You may want to take something for an easy breakfast on your first morning in your new space. If you're taking cereal, remember you'll need milk, bowls, and spoons.

***Take medications with you***. Do not pack medications in any box, and definitely, *do not send them with the movers*. If the unexpected happens, you'll have your medications as needed when you take them with you.

## Unpacking

Full-service moving companies offer unpacking as well as packing. Of course, this is an added cost, but one you may find very helpful.

- **Advantages of Moving Company Unpacking:**

  o All boxes and containers are unpacked, and items are put away in cupboards and closets on the day of your move. The only exception is wall hangings; these are unpacked but not hung on the walls.

  o All packing boxes and packing materials are removed when empty.

  o You save days, and possibly weeks, of unpacking and putting things away; your new home is live-in ready on your first day.

- **Disadvantages of Moving Company Unpacking**

  o You may not find things where you expect them to be.

  o It adds to the expense of your move.

One important factor for using the unpacking option may be how able you are to do the work. If you're moving to Assisted Living, this service may be provided. No matter where you're moving, you may want to have your apartment live-in ready, knowing you can rearrange things when you're more familiar with your new routine.

# Insurance

There are two kinds of insurance offered by moving companies:

- Full value protection means your mover is liable for the total replacement value of any lost or damaged items in your shipment.

- Released value protection means you pay no additional cost, but you'll only receive up to 60 cents per pound for an item.[36]

If you select released value from your mover, you may want to buy movers insurance from a third party. But, before buying any insurance, check your homeowner's policy to see if you're already covered." [37]

If you have antique furniture and/or collectibles, you may want to insure them through third-party insurance. They'll need to be appraised for value in case of damage or loss. If the antiques are family heirlooms, they may be irreplaceable, and you'll need to decide if your item is lost or damaged, if you'll accept a similar item or cash for replacement. If your items are more sentimental than valuable, you'll want to decide whether it's worthwhile to pay the extra cost of full-value insurance.

When selecting which insurance option to take, remember the decision applies to everything you are sending with the movers. Which insurance to take is totally a personal decision based on your sense of the value of your household goods. If you have one extremely valuable item, you may consider hiring a specialized mover for that piece.

## Choosing the Right Moving Company for You

Compare costs and services for different moving companies, taking into consideration what is included in the bid. The form at the end of this chapter makes it easier to compare companies.

The agreed-upon cost, specific services, date and time for the move, and any packing, should be in writing, and the contract should be signed by the company representative as well as by you.

# Step Three: Moving Day

If you're using Senior Movers, they can handle the details of your move. Otherwise, you'll be in charge. Be ready at the designated time. If there are items not to be moved, be sure they're marked appropriately. Someone should be at your house while the movers are there and then at your new home when they arrive. Coordination, if you are moving a long distance, may take more planning.

Have your floor plan available, so that when your furniture arrives, you can tell the movers exactly where you want each item placed. If you're doing the unpacking, make sure boxes go into the appropriate rooms. The drawers from your bedroom chests are usually transported with everything in them, so you'll have immediate access to those clothes.

If the movers are working as mealtime approaches, you may want to purchase sandwiches or pizza for them. This isn't necessary, but a nice gesture. You may also want to tip the crew when they finish if they've done a good job.

If the movers have unpacked, you're ready to settle into your new home. If you'll be doing the unpacking, the first thing to open is your "ESSENTIAL" box(es). Make your bed, put your towels in the bathroom, and plug in your coffee pot. Your new home may be a maze of boxes, but you're ready to spend a comfortable night.

Over the next week or so, you'll open all the boxes and put things where you want them. When you dispose of the last box, you can give a sigh of relief, you're fully moved into your new home.

# Step Four: Change of Address Notifications

There are many companies, agencies, and people you'll need to notify of your change of address. *A list of the most common is found at the end of this chapter*; you also may have others more unique to your own situation. You can check each one off as you complete it.

# Summary

Moving requires a lot of planning and preparation. You must decide whether to keep, sell, or rent your house. Choosing a moving company and deciding how much of the preparation and unpacking will be done by you and/or by the moving company takes time and thought. Deciding on the insurance needed is important. During the period when you're preparing for the move, you'll also need to notify all relevant companies, agencies, and people of your change of address.

Although it may seem like the moving process will never end, when you're settled in your new home, you'll quickly forget all the issues that seemed monumental at the time.

# Moving Company Bids
## Work Sheet

**Name of Company** _____

**Telephone Number** _____

**Agent** _____

**Date** _____

**Services included:**

Packing                           Yes               No

                                  Cost      $_____

Unpacking                         Yes               No

                                  Cost      $_____

**Insurance:**

Coverage:      Full Value Protection _____

               Cost            $_____

               Released Value Protection _____

               Home Owners Insurance Coverage     Yes      No

**Total Moving Cost**                      $_____

Price determined by weight                 Yes              No

Price determined by in-home assessment     Yes              No

# Address Changes

## Updating Your Life
## Work Sheet

- **Mail** ___

  Obtain a *Change of Address* form at the Post Office

  Be aware that the time when mail will be forwarded is limited, and only first-class mail will be forwarded unless you specifically request magazines, catalogs and flyers.

- **All sources for checks you receive regularly but aren't directly deposited to your bank account** _____

- **Credit cards** _____

- **Social Security** _____

- **Bank and/or Credit Union accounts** _____

- **Driver's License/Car Registration/
  Handicapped Placard** _____

- **Voter Registration** _____

- **Insurance companies**

  o *Car* _____

  o *Home Insurance (Cancel)* _____

  o *Renter's/CCRC Insurance (Purchase)* _____

  o *Whole Life Insurance* _____

- o   *Medical/Medicare* _____
- o   *Long Term Health Insurance* _____
- o   *Other* _____

- **All companies where you have credit accounts you're using**

  - o   *Department stores* _____
  - o   *On-line Retailers* _____
  - o   *Other* _____

- **Cancel Home Utilities**

  - o   *Gas* _____
  - o   *Electric* _____
  - o   *Water* _____
  - o   *Sewer* _____
  - o   *Trash Removal* _____
  - o   *Landline telephone* _____
  - o   *Cable and/or Satellite* _____
  - o   *Home Security System* _____

- **Newspaper(s)** _____
- **Medical Alert System** _____
- **Mobile Phone Plan** _____
- **Financial advisor** _____

- **Attorney** _____

- **Doctors/Dentists** _____

- **All stocks, bonds, or securities not managed by a financial agency** _____

- **Family and friends** _____

- **Magazines and catalogues** _____

- **Library card** _____

- **Landscaping, Pool Maintenance, Snow Removal** _____

# You've Made It! Jump in and Enjoy!

## Your New Life Begins

The movers are gone and you're standing in your new home. You're surrounded by familiar furniture, but it may look strange and unfamiliar in the new setting. No matter whether the movers unpacked your boxes or they're stacked everywhere, you'll be tired.

Before you do one more thing, sit down in your living room and take a break. Have a glass of wine or a cup of tea, and toast your new life. You've done it! You've researched, made a lot of difficult decisions and done the hard work of moving. Yes, there still may be all those boxes to unpack and put away and unfinished business to deal with, but the hardest work is behind you.

After your break, if you're doing the unpacking yourself, open your "Essentials" box, hang up the towels and make your bed. You may want to go to dinner in the dining room, stay in and have a makeshift dinner using the contents of your ice chest, or even call a food delivery service. It's your choice.

Don't unpack anything other than your "Essentials" box and your ice chest the first night. If the movers unpacked for you, you don't need to locate anything other than those things you need immediately. Moving is exhausting and you have plenty of time to unpack and settle in. Spend the evening relaxing. Go to bed early. Tomorrow is another day and your boxes will wait.

# Your First Week or Two

Hopefully, you had a good night's sleep and are up and ready to go on your first full day in your new home. If breakfast is part of your meal plan, you may want to go to the dining room to eat. Or, you may prefer to have breakfast in your apartment.

This is the week (or two) you'll spend unpacking, getting acquainted with your new home, meeting your neighbors and others, and start learning your way around your new community.

For those who had the movers unpack, now is the time to look in the kitchen and other storage areas and perhaps move some things around so they're more convenient for you. For those with boxes waiting to be unpacked, it's time to roll up your sleeves and get to work.

## Unpacking

You may want to start with the kitchen and bathroom boxes as you may want to use the contents sooner. The kitchen is the room that takes the longest to unpack and put away. Before you start, look around and think about where you might want to place the essentials.

What will go on the countertops? Is there enough room to include all those small appliances you normally keep on the countertops? Can you reach all the shelves? If some are too high to reach easily, you may want to leave them unused or put seldom-used items on them. If they're adjustable, you may want to resize them.

Put the things you use every day on the most accessible shelves. Although you can always rearrange your kitchen cabinets, most of us never do, so take your time. If you don't have enough kitchen shelf space for everything, you may want to reconsider whether you need everything you brought. Or, you may want to purchase a free-standing cabinet, perhaps with wheels, to provide additional storage and counter space.

Don't spend all day every day unpacking. Yes, you want to get settled as soon as possible, but there's no point exhausting yourself. Take breaks and get out a little, even if it's only to check your mail and go to dinner.

## Organizing and Decorating

If you brought books to donate to your community's library, take them to the library. Not only will you get the books out of your space, but you may have a chance to meet a library volunteer and learn more about how your library functions.

If you need help connecting your TV and computer to the cable and Wi-Fi, put in a work order for maintenance. They can probably take care of it quickly. Make sure all large appliances work. Even though your new home was totally redone before your arrival, there may be glitches and you want to take care of them as soon as possible.

By the end of your first full week or two, you should be pretty well settled. The last thing to do is hang your pictures and wall art. Now that your furniture is in place, you can figure out where you want to put each piece of art. Get them all out of their packing boxes and lay them on the floor.

One-by-one, take each to a potential site and hold it up in the spot where it might go. Don't be limited to thinking it has to go in the same room where it went before. When you find the spot where you think it looks best, lean it against the wall or on a piece of furniture under that spot.

When you've put each item in a tentative spot, you may have some items left over. Put them aside for the time being. You may also want to switch pieces around as you continue to think about them.

When you feel confident you've found the right place for each, it's time to hang them. Be sure to know the community guidelines for hanging pictures.

Correctly centering and hanging pictures straight is not easy. For heavier items, finding a wall stud is essential if you're using picture nails. If all this is more than you want to tackle yourself, you might call on a family member who's willing to help or maintenance may provide this service. Another option is to hire a handyman; some communities have someone you can call.

# Extras that May Make Your Life Easier

You may want to purchase a few extras that will make your life even easier or more comfortable.

## Shopping Cart

You'll be going shopping from time to time, and you'll need to get your purchases from your car or the community's transportation to your home. Carrying armloads of packages is not convenient, comfortable, or even possible sometimes.

If you have a central laundry area, a cart is ideal for transporting your clothes back and forth as well. You can put hangers on the handle and folded clothes inside. Some carts come with an inside cloth cover that can be used for transporting your clean laundry.

If you live in an apartment and order online, you may need to take your packages and boxes from the front desk to your apartment. You can even use the cart to transport your pet in its carrier.

## Wireless Door Bell

For those with hearing issues, a door bell may be a necessity; for others, it's still helpful. Widely available in stores and online, they are easily installed.

## Sliding Kitchen Drawers

For many of us, getting things out of the low kitchen cabinets is difficult. It's hard to see what's in the back and even harder to reach the items stored there if your cabinets don't come with sliding drawers. These drawers make all the difference in how much these cabinets can be used. Again, they are widely available in stores and online. Some are quite easy to install, but as they are down low, you may want to have someone else do the installation.

## Bathroom Caddy

If your shower doesn't come with built-in storage for soap, shampoo, etc., you may want to purchase a bathroom caddy. Again, these are readily available and fairly inexpensive. The best type for a rental apartment requires no drilling. There are two kinds, the first is free standing; the other is attached to the wall with an adhesive that can be removed without leaving a mark. It's very easy to install these yourself.

## Carts and Shelves

A cart with wheels, or legs can be useful in many areas and can be purchased to fit your available space. A cart in the kitchen provides extra storage space as well as extra counter space. This may be the ideal spot for your coffee pot or other often used small appliance.

Freestanding carts or cabinets, with drawers, are useful in the bathroom if you don't have enough storage. You can also buy bathroom shelves to store towels and supplies above the toilet or on a wall. These can be attractive as well as utilitarian.

You'll need some sort of laundry hamper or basket for your dirty clothes. If you have a laundry area in your apartment, you may have room nearby for a small cart to hold your soap and other laundry supplies.

## Shower Curtain Magnets

If you have a walk-in shower with a shower curtain, you'll need shower curtain magnets to keep the floor outside the shower dry. Their weight holds the curtain in place and keeps the water inside where it belongs. These are small round discs that you place near the bottom of the shower curtain. One disc goes on each side of the curtain and the magnetic power holds them together.

# Start Living Your New Life

During your first weeks, while you're getting settled, you'll probably begin meeting your neighbors. If you can remember the names of a few of your closest neighbors, great. If you don't, it's not a problem. Everyone understands how overwhelming it is to meet so many new people. As time goes on, you'll get to know and remember more residents. If you're given a name tag, wear it. It will help others remember your name better. (Hopefully, they'll wear theirs as well.)

If you've been given a handbook or other information about life in your new community, skim it and read any parts that will be helpful as you get settled. Keep it handy as you will refer to it from time to time for pertinent information.

Start going to all meals included in your plan, every day. It may feel intimidating to walk into the dining room if you don't know anyone but do it anyway. If there's a host or hostess, they may seat you. If you're invited to sit with others, accept the invitation; it's a great way to get acquainted. Each community has its own customs, and you'll soon learn what those are in your community. The wait staff is a good source of information.

Get a copy of the current activities calendar and decide what looks interesting to you. Choose a few activities and/or programs each day and go to them.

If possible, at least several times a week, commit to going to an exercise class. "Physical activity can help you think, learn, problem-solve, and enjoy an emotional balance. It can improve memory and reduce anxiety or depression.

Regular physical activity can also reduce your risk of cognitive decline, including dementia. One study found that cognitive decline is almost twice as common among adults who are inactive compared to those who are active."[38]

What activities appeal to you? Do you like games? There's sure to be a game, or several, you'll enjoy. Maybe you'd like to participate in an arts and crafts class or a discussion group; if so, try them out. Attend programs, both for information and entertainment.

A good way to get to know other residents is to sign up for an off-campus dining excursion. Because you'll be sitting at a table with other residents, you'll have an hour or more to talk and get to know them better.

Before you know it, if you're making an effort to get out and about, you'll find that some residents who were complete strangers a few weeks ago are becoming your friends. You'll find you feel comfortable in your new routine and very glad you made the decision to move. You did all the hard work; it was worth it.

**You're home!**

## Summary

Once you've physically moved in, it's time to create your new life. Start by placing your furniture and accessories in an arrangement that feels comfortable to you. When you've put everything in its place and hung your wall art, your new home will reflect who you are. Purchase any small items needed for the finishing touches and to provide additional storage.

Get involved in the daily life of your new community. Join classes, attend programs, and eat in the dining room. Day by day, you'll get to know the other residents and begin to feel more and more at home. If you're like many of us, you won't even be nostalgic for your old house. It's part of your past and you're living a fulfilling life in the present.

# Tying Up Loose Ends

## The Final Steps

You've moved and are settling into your senior living community. There may be some loose ends that need to be addressed before you're totally free from the past. You may need to sell or rent your house, get rid of a storage unit, invest the equity from your house, change your medical providers, and/or revisit and update some legal documents. If you moved to a new state, there will be more to do.

# Financial Issues

## Your House

If you decided to wait to sell or rent your house, it's time to get it on the market or listed with a management company. The longer it remains empty, the more it may lose value. A broken water pipe or leaking water heater, if not discovered quickly, can cause extensive damage. Even normal deterioration will eventually become evident and reduce the value of your house. It's like an albatross around your neck—weighing you down with thoughts of what needs to be done. Take the first step and act.

## Storage Unit

If you rented a storage unit, start cleaning it out and either move things you want to your new apartment or donate them. You want to be finished with the storage unit as soon as possible. (Remember, you promised yourself you wouldn't keep it longer than six months!) After a couple of weeks, you have a pretty good idea of what you can use and what you can't. Go through the boxes and be ruthless with your decisions. Even if you dispose of something you later need, it probably won't cost the rent of a month of storage to replace.

## Remaining Equity

If you didn't use all the equity you received from your house; it's time to invest it. You'll want to leave a balance readily available as a cushion for any extra costs or anticipated expenses during the next year but for the remainder, make an appointment with your financial advisor and move ahead. You can decide on your risk level, but even a low interest rate is better than you'll earn if you leave the money in a checking account.

# Medical Providers

If you can continue to easily see your health care providers after you've moved, there's no need to change. However, if you're moving farther away from the community where you lived previously, you'll need to change all your providers, including those you may not see on a regular basis. You'll also want to know what hospital is closest to your new home.

If you need to change your medical provider, the first step is to call your insurance company for a list of primary doctors they accept. Make sure those recommended are currently accepting new patients.

Talk to other residents to get feedback about their doctors. If they've had good experiences with specific doctors, put a checkmark by the name of that provider. Read online profiles to see if those recommended are board-certified and/or have specific qualifications. Read any reviews available. Remember most people only post reviews when they are unsatisfied with the service they received, and positive reviews could be posted by friends of the provider. Use your judgement about how useful the reviews are.

Make your next appointment with a primary doctor you think may be a good fit for you. If you're satisfied after your first appointment, they can refer you to specialists. If you're not satisfied, schedule another provider for your next appointment. Don't take too long to decide; you want to become established with your new team as soon as possible.

## Legal Documents

All elders should have five legal documents; a Living Will, a POLST, a Power of Attorney, a Medical Power of Attorney, and a Will. If you already have these documents, you may need to amend them to reflect your current information. If you don't have them, now is a good time to get them.

### Living Will

Your *Living Will* lets your doctors know how you want to be treated if you are seriously ill and incapable of making and communicating your wishes. If you currently have a *Living Will*, it is transferable,[39] but needs to be updated with your new address and any information that has changed. You'll want to give an updated copy to your new doctors, the hospital, your family, and the person with your *Power of Medical Attorney.*

### POLST (Also Known as a POST, MOLST, COLST or MOST in Some States)

The *Provider Orders for Life-Sustaining Treatment* is more commonly known as a POLST. It is more comprehensive than a DNR

(Do Not Resuscitate) and is a document every senior should have. It communicates your end-of-life wishes related to emergency medical services. Although the POLST is transferrable in most states, it's a good idea to check with your doctor about the status in your new state.[40] Keep your old POLST on the refrigerator (where the EMTs are trained to look) until you update it.

## Power of Attorney

Your *Power of Attorney* designates someone to act as your agent in certain situations. A *Power of Attorney* document is accepted in all states; however, each state has its own rules and requirements. It is better to create a new document that matches the style used in your new state.[41] You may also want to change your designated *Power of Attorney* to someone who lives close to your new location. Consult an attorney if you're updating your P*ower of Attorney*

## Power of Medical Attorney

A *Power of Medical Attorney* is not the same as a *Power of Attorney*. Again, this document is extremely important if you need to go to a hospital or care center and cannot advocate for yourself. Your designated agent needs to be someone in close proximity in case of an emergency. Again, consult an attorney if you're updating your *Power of Medical Attorney.*

## Trusts and Wills

You may need to update your *Trust* or *Will* if the disposition of your house or any other assets have changed. This is a fairly easy correction. Check with your attorney to see if you can change it yourself.

When you've tied up all your loose ends, you're ready to completely embrace your new life as an elder.

## Summary

Moving during our elder years requires more than just relocating to another home. By this time, we probably have at least several doctors and will need to replace all of them if we're moving very far. Finding new health providers takes time and effort, but it's extremely important so you can build a relationship before there's an emergency. When your house is sold or rented, you've gotten rid of your storage unit, and you've invested any remaining equity, your finances are in place. Revising or redoing legal papers ensures everything is in place if or when they're needed. You're now able to fully enjoy your new life with enthusiasm and peace of mind.

The End

# Footnote References

[1] https://www.ncbi.nlm.nih.gov/books/NBK235450/

[2] https://www.sciencealert.com/our-bodies-age-in-three-separate-shifts-according-new-blood-tests

[3] https://www.agingcare.com/articles/legally-force-move-to-assisted-living-155888.htm

[4] https://www.pewresearch.org/short-reads/2024/01/09/us-centenarian-population-is-projected-to-quadruple-over-the-next-30-years/

[5] https://www.nia.nih.gov/news/social-isolation-loneliness-older-people-pose-health-risks

[6] https://www.fbi.gov/how-we-can-help-you/scams-and-safety/common-frauds-and-scams/elder-fraud

[7] https://www.aarp.org/caregiving/basics/info-2022/housing-options.html

[8] https://www.aarp.org/caregiving/basics/info-2017/continuing-care-retirement-communities.html

[9] https://dickinsonlaw.psu.edu/sites/default/files/2022-05/Pearson-Here%E2%80%99s-how-continuing-care-retirement-communities-work-and-why-some-go-bankrupt.pdf

[10] https://www.wsj.com/articles/retirees-life-savings-can-vanish-in-continuing-care-bankruptcies-dfe55c7d

[11] https://www.nic.org/news-press/senior-housing-residents-live-longer-than-counterparts-living-in-the-community/

[12] https://www.501c3.org/what-is-a-501c3/

[13] https://www.seniorliving.org/continuing-care-retirement-communities/

[14] https://www.seniorliving.org/care/cost/affordable/

[15] https://www.seniorliving.org/care/cost/affordable/

[16] https://www.ncoa.org/article/a-guide-to-section-202-low-Income-housing-for-older-adults/

[17] https://www.va.gov/health-care/about-va-health-benefits/long-term-care/

[18] https://health.usnews.com/senior-care/articles/levels-of-care-for-the-elderly

[19] https://northstarsa.com/senior-housing-vs-senior-living/

[20] https://seniorservicesofamerica.com/blog/what-does-assisted-living-provide-for-residents/

[21] https://www.caitlin-morgan.com/ada-compliance-nursing-homes-assisted-living-facilities/#:~:text=Be%20designed%20so%20that%20all,light%20characters%20on%20light%20backgrounds.

[22] https://residentialassistedlivingacademy.com/the-ultimate-guide-to-assisted-living-staff/

[23] https://www.ncoa.org/adviser/local-care/memory-care/

[24] https://www.nm.org/healthbeat/healthy-tips/emotional-health/music-as-medicine-alzheimers-dementia

[25] https://www.uhhospitals.org/health-information/health-and-wellness-library/article/adult-diseases-and-conditions-v1/skilled-nursing-facility-snf

[26] https://www.seniorliving.org/custodial-care/

[27] https://www.whereyoulivematters.org/resources/life-senior-living-community

[28] https://www.hud.gov/program_offices/fair_housing_equal_opp/fair_housing_act_housing_older_persons#_What_Are_the

[29] https://www.hansonbridgett.com/sites/default/files/sitecore/Files/Publications/2016-1-pag-seniors-housing-guide.pdf

[30] https://www.washingtonpost.com/business/2023/12/17/assisted-

living-laws-rules-states/

[31] https://seniorservicesofamerica.com/blog/alcohol-and-assisted-living/

[32] https://pmc.ncbi.nlm.nih.gov/articles/PMC6388774/

[33] https://www.seniorliving.org/continuing-care-retirement-communities/

[34] https://www.franketobeyjones.com/senior-living-contracts-explained/

[35] https://www.bankrate.com/mortgages/bridge-loan/

[36] https://www.fmcsa.dot.gov/consumer-protection/protect-your-move/how-do-i-insure-my-belongings-during-moveare

[37] Ibid

[38] https://www.cdc.gov/physical-activity/features/boost-brain-health.html

[39] https://order.nia.nih.gov/sites/default/files/2023-04/nia-advance-care-planning.pdf

[40] https://www.americanbar.org/groups/law_aging/publications/bifoc al/vol_36/issue_1_october2014/polst_legislative_comparison_and_u pdate/

[41] https://www.elderlawanswers.com/is-a-power-of-attorney-valid-in-another-state-15293

www.ingramcontent.com/pod-product-compliance
Lightning Source LLC
Chambersburg PA
CBHW071020120626
46546CB00003B/1179

* 9 7 8 1 9 6 8 9 6 6 0 4 1 *